30 Days to
Total Brain Health®

A Whole Month's Worth of Daily Tips

to

Boost Your Memory

And Build

Better Brain Power

Cynthia R. Green, Ph.D.

President of Memory Arts LLC
and Founding Director of the
Memory Enhancement Program
Mount Sinai School of Medicine

Also By Cynthia R. Green, Ph.D.

Total Memory Workout: 8 Easy Steps to Maximum Memory Fitness

Through the Seasons: An Activity Book for Memory-Challenged Adults and Caregivers

Brainpower Game Plan: Food, Moves and Games to Clear Brain Fog, Boost Memory and Age-Proof Your Mind in 4 Weeks!

The Good Thinking Kit

Want to know more about these products?
Visit www.totalbrainhealth.com/store

"Three cheers for Dr. Green!" – *Jeanette K., student*

Get ready to make the move to better brain health!

In this remarkably effective, scientifically-grounded plan, Dr. Cynthia Green, a clinical psychologist and one of the country's most notable experts on brain health, has just what you need to start on the road to better brain fitness. Based on her multi-dimensional, integrated Total Brain Health® model, Dr. Green has laid out 30 days of simple tips certain to boost your everyday memory and reduce your dementia risk. In just 10 minutes a day or less, you'll use Dr. Green's unique Body|Mind|Spirit approach to build your brainpower in ways you'd never imagined, such as:

- **Get Some Phone Game**. *Learn why playing around with your phone can be good for your brain.*
- **Doodle**! *Did you know that doodling is good for your noodle? Find out why.*
- **Tap a Tune**. *Spend some time banging out your own personal beat and boosting your brain power as a result.*

"After practicing several of the techniques I see measurable memory improvement. People are now commenting on my great memory and I am apologizing less!" – *Michelle B.*

"One reason for taking the course was because I started a new job and knew I had weeks of major intense training with tons of information to remember. I've been passing all the tests and retaining the information – today I received an award for knowing the company's vision statement which I had memorized." – *Lisa M.*

"After years of placing the blame on age, Dr. Green has helped me to understand I do not have to stand by helplessly but rather can direct my own course of action in overcoming memory glitches." – *Doris K.*

30 Days to Total Brain Health®

PUBLISHING HISTORY

Memory Arts LLC Trade paperback | September 2011

ISBN 978-0-578-08718-4

MEMORY ARTS LLC

P.O. BOX 3386

MEMORIAL STATION

UPPER MONTCLAIR, N.J. 07043

www.totalbrainhealth.com

PRINTED IN THE UNITED STATES OF AMERICA

To Josh, Zach, Jonah and Hannah
Who make it all worth remembering!

and

In Memory of Beverly Jablons
Who left us many memories too short

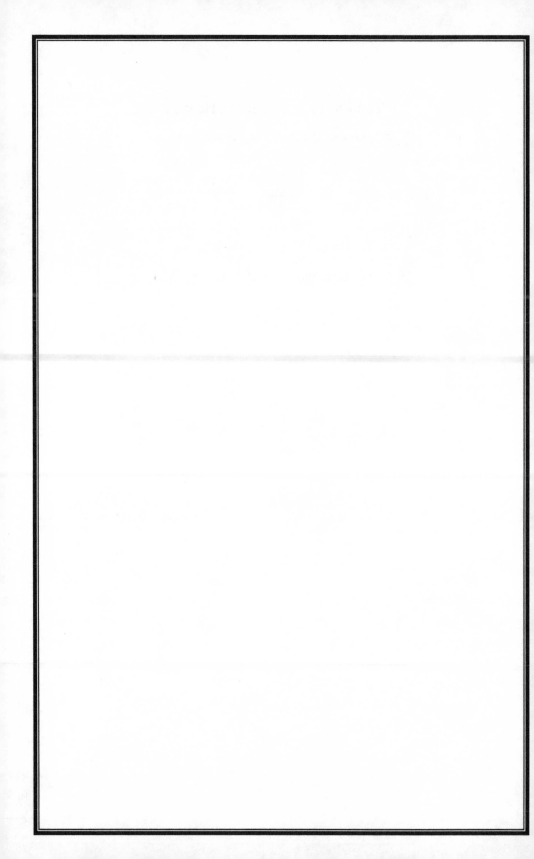

Introduction

What is brain health? In truth, many of us aren't sure what brain health means exactly, or what we have to do to achieve better brain health. Do we need to do more to keep our brains busy? Should we take up a new language, or start doing the daily crossword? What really makes the difference when it comes to staying sharp and lowering our risk for a memory disorder down the road?

As an expert in memory fitness and brain health, the best part of my job is teaching people what brain health is all about. Taking away the mystery of what we mean by "brain health" is part of the reason I like what I do. Some of the research on brain health can be a bit surprising (for example did you know that having a sense of purpose has been associated with a reduced dementia risk?), while other findings support good, old-fashioned medical advice that is familiar to us all. In fact, chances are you have already started on the path to better brain health without even knowing it.

This book is the result of a program I ran on my website over January 2011. Originally the idea was to provide folks with fun, quick and easy things they could do in about 10 minutes a day over one month as a way of kicking off a brain healthy year. As I wrote each day's "tip," I realized that there was so much to say about each one, for example in explaining the science behind what might seem like a quirky suggestion, or making a tip easier to try. What was supposed to be limited to 140 characters (a familiar limitation to those of you that "tweet") became a bit lengthier. And before I knew it, another book was in the works.

What is Brain Health?

What do we mean when we refer to "brain health?" At its most basic, the term refers literally to the physiological health of the brain as an organ. However, most of us also use the term to include the ways in which that underlying physical state is expressed. We "see" our brain's health reflected in how we function day to day, including how well we are able to attend, learn and remember. In addition, our brain health impacts our ability to stay vital and independent, especially as we age. Finally, the term brain health is often used to denote something about our risk for dementia, and what we can do to manage, to the degree that we can, that risk. These aspects of brain health are in great part expressions of each other. One would be quite challenged to stay self-reliant and pursue passions in later life without well-preserved intellectual function. Yet it is important that we appreciate all these facets of brain health to fully understand its meaning.

Achieving Brain Health: The Total Brain Health® Model

One of my main goals as an educator in the field of brain health is to translate the latest research into sensible strategies anyone can use to improve intellectual performance and lower dementia risk. We have made remarkable strides in understanding how the brain works and what it needs to stay healthy. But putting these discoveries to work means more than simply doing crossword puzzles or playing chess. I arrived at the Total Brain Health® model as a way of turning this complex new science into a practical blueprint for enhancing brain fitness. I call this approach Total Brain Health® because it improves mental acuity and helps maintain cognitive vitality by addressing <u>all</u> of the ways our overall health influences brain fitness. The three dimensions of the Total Brain Health® Model are:

- *Body*: Our physical well-being is critical to healthy brain functioning, underscoring the importance of lifestyle choices such as diet and exercise.

- *Mind*: Intellectual well-being through mentally stimulating activities that challenge skills, stretch our mental capacity, and teach us memory strategies is essential for brain health.

- *Spirit*: Staving off the damaging effects of stress and other negative emotions, while filling our lives with satisfying personal relationships, offers surprising benefits for the brain.

Total Brain Health® targets each of these essential areas with interventions that are proven to enhance daily intellectual performance and reduce the risk for dementia. The 30 Day Program contained in this book reflects this philosophy, offering a chance to taste each day something better you can do for your brain across the whole spectrum of brain wellness.

May the next 30 days get you off on a great start to better brain health. You will be trying new things, seeing the same things in a slightly different way, or learning a new way of doing something you've done forever. Whatever your experience, I have no doubt that you will come out of it with smarter brain habits and on the road to your own Total Brain Health® experience.

Here's to many happy memories!

Cynthia R. Green, Ph.D.

NOTES FOR DAY 1

DAY 1

Get Physical!

Welcome to Day One! To kick off the month, let's begin with one of the most "tried and true" things we can do to boost our brain's well-being -- aerobic exercise. Recent research shows that regular aerobic exercise can:

- Improve your memory and other skills, such as attention, processing speed and executive control, which matter to daily intellectual performance.
- Significantly decrease your risk for dementia.
- Significantly reduce your risk for or be an important part of managing medical conditions that in turn increase your risk for dementia, such as obesity, diabetes, and hypertension.

Start today on the road to better brain health by boosting your exercise time. *Get at least 30 minutes of exercise several days a week.* Even brisk walking has been proven to be beneficial to brain health. Make it easier to stick with your exercise plan by penciling in time to work out, finding an exercise buddy, or setting clear exercise goals with built-in rewards.

What a great way to get started.

NOTES FOR DAY 2

DAY 2

Play Online

Today's tip gives you a chance to boost your brain power by taking 10 minutes a day to play. What could be more fun than that?

Research has shown that we can better maintain intellectual skills, such as attention, speed, executive control and memory (all of which can change as we age) by giving them a good "work out." One of the best ways to keep these skills challenged is by playing games against the clock, since timed activities force us to focus, think fast and be nimble in our approach.

Games we play online tend to be timed and can give our brains a terrific skills challenge. Look at free games on sites such as www.miniclip.com (Sushi Go Round is still one of my favorites), or check out some of the brain fitness software products on the market such as Lumosity or Happy Neuron (many of these sites now offer games you can download to your phone or tablet). Prevention Magazine's website offers brain games, as do several other sites, including the AARP.

So go ahead today and play online – It's fun, it's free, and it's good for your brain.

NOTES FOR DAY 3

DAY 3

Tap a Tune

Today's better brain health tip is sure to get you moving to a different beat. Go ahead and make up a little tune by tapping your fingers on your table or desktop (the actual desktop, not the computer, though I guess you could make up a tune using those computer keys if you are so inclined).

Your tune can be as short or long, simple or complex, though I would suggest going for more than just one "note." Tapping a tune will challenge your brain to think about the world in a slightly different way, and get you to coordinate your movement, auditory and memory skills. Imagine -- all that in just a few minutes today.

Who knows, you could even come up with your own personal theme song!

NOTES FOR DAY 4

DAY 4

Learn About Memory Loss

Today's tip challenges you to learn a bit more about memory loss. I am often asked what memory loss is all about, and when someone should worry about changes in their memory. Here's your chance to take a few minutes and find some answers to your own questions about memory.

The Alzheimer's Association is the leading non-profit organization for information and support for those concerned about memory loss. Many don't realize what a wonderful resource the Alzheimer's Association is for general information about memory health, but their website actually covers everything from memory changes that can come with age (including some terrific brain health advice), early symptoms to look for, as well as the how's and why's of evaluation for memory loss.

So take a few minutes today to check out the Alzheimer's Association website at www.alz.org — it's a good thing to do for your brain.

NOTES FOR DAY 5

DAY 5

Do a Word Search

Today's tip will get you to re-work a word. Take the words below and see how many other words you can come up with, using the letters of the original word. This "word search" game gives your brain a boost by getting you to be more nimble in your thinking and shift your usual way of seeing things. Want to up the challenge? Give yourself 2 minutes per word.

RESOLUTION

SUFFICIENT

BENEFICENCE

SYNAPSE

PROPAGATION

Happy searching!

NOTES FOR DAY 6

DAY 6

Check Your Blood Pressure

Today's tip comes right out of the medical textbooks: Take a few minutes today to check your blood pressure.

Hypertension, or high blood pressure, when not controlled by lifestyle or medication, can seriously increase your risk for stroke. Stroke is, after all, a brain injury, the leading cause of disability in the U.S. and a major cause of memory loss (as well as the third leading cause of death).

You can have your blood pressure checked at most pharmacies, many of which have a blood pressure machine available. If your pressure seems higher than usual, follow up with your doctor. Hypertension can readily be managed, reducing your stroke risk.

Want to reduce your risk for stroke? A 2008 study from the Harvard School of Public Health found that we could reduce our risk for stroke by up to 80% by leading a brain healthy lifestyle, including regular exercise, a healthy diet, maintaining a healthy weight and not smoking.

Now that's something to think about.

NOTES FOR DAY 7

DAY 7

Color Your World

Today's the day to bring out your inner artist (even if you haven't so much as scribbled since you were 8).

New or different activities such as coloring, even if we do them just briefly, refresh our attention, get us to try new (or rarely used) skills, and challenge us to see the world in a different way.

What do you need to fulfill today's tip? Just go get a set of crayons, markers, or colored pencils and spend some time doodling, drawing, or sketching. You can even purchase an abstract coloring book (you can find them online) to help you color away the minutes. Have kids? Share this activity and have fun together.

NOTES FOR DAY 8

DAY 8

Volunteer

Want to do something that's good for others and good for your brain? Look today for ways you can volunteer.

Studies have shown that folks who volunteer are healthier overall, including on measures that gauge everyday intellectual well-being. Volunteering also gives you a way to stay intellectually and socially engaged, both of which have been associated with a reduced risk for major memory impairment.

There are certainly many ways and places for you to volunteer your time within your community, no matter how much (or little!) time you may have. Look to sites such as www.volunteermatch.org for ideas and resources.

NOTES FOR DAY 9

DAY 9

Tell a Tale

Today's tip will rev up your own inner storyteller. Take one of the "story starters" below and weave a tale of your own.

This short exercise is certain to get your creative juices going and give you a great way to challenge your mind in a new and different way. Research has shown that staying intellectually engaged may lower our dementia risk, so go ahead and start telling your tale.

Try starting your story with one of the following lines, or beginning with one of your own:

"As she walked along the narrow path, Martha came upon .... "

" Little did I suspect that ... "

"The noises of the night rarely disturbed Roger's sleep, yet that night the ... "

If you are inspired by today's tip, check out websites such as www.dailywritingtips.com for more tips on taking pen to paper.

NOTES FOR DAY 10

DAY 10

Try Something Fun!

Hey folks, it's Day 10! Why not start off with a bit of fun that's also good for your brain?

Today's tip? Try something a bit silly that lifts your spirits. Why? Well, why not?! Every once in a while we need something to lighten our mood. Emotional distress, such as feeling blue, feeling anxious, or just plain feeling stressed, take a toll on our memory by making it harder for us to be focused.

Let's face it, its distracting to feel down! So try something that makes your spirits soar and put a smile on your face.

If you need some inspiration, try putting on some favorite dance tunes and strut your stuff a bit – that always puts a smile on my face!

NOTES FOR DAY 11

DAY 11

Jump Some Jacks

Today's tip brings us back to basics. As we learned on Day #1 (and which you definitely remember), aerobic exercise is one of the best things we can do for our brain. For today, you're going to jive up your brain by doing some jumping jacks.

You DO remember jumping jacks, don't you? Jumping jacks are a simple calisthenics exercise you can do standing in place that can quickly get your blood pumping. If you need a refresher course, just look on the internet for instructions.

So simply stand up and do a set of 10. Or 20. Do several sets over the course of today. Your brain will once again thank you.

Happy jumping!

NOTES FOR DAY 12

DAY 12

Learn a Poem

Today's tip offers you two brain health challenges! Reading poetry gets our mind out of its "box" and is a wonderful source of intellectual challenge and pleasure. Memorizing a poem offers a different kind of brain workout, honing our rote memorization skills, which we used quite a bit in school but may not exercise frequently in "real life."

So your task for today is to find a poem and spend a few minutes (or more) reading and musing it over. Then try memorizing it, so that you can keep it with you always and even share it with others.

Need a great resource for poems? Try www.poets.org, the website of the Academy of American Poets. You can even sign up for their "Poem a Day" program and get a poem sent to your inbox each day. The poems sent are usually seasonal, and range from well-loved poems to newly published ones. I've subscribed for several months now, and it's one of my very favorite things to receive.

Found a poem you love? Share it with someone.

NOTES FOR DAY 13

| |
| |
| |
| |
| |
| |
| |
| |
| |
| |
| |
| |
| |
| |
| |
| |
| |
| |
| |
| |

DAY 13

The Honorable Opposition

Today's tip asks you to open your mind. Often we fall into the rut of only listening to information and opinions that reaffirm the beliefs we already hold, be it in our political, philosophical or personal lives. Listening to the opposite point of view can get us to re-think our positions (though not necessarily change them!), giving us a chance to engage our minds in a way we may not have done in quite a while and perhaps even see things from another's point of view.

Spend some time today tuning in to TV, radio stations or reading articles that hold the opposite political point of view to your own. Try talking about what you read with friends or family, seeing if you can even hold the counter position in your discussions.

NOTES FOR DAY 14

DAY 14

Take a Yoga Break

Today's tip is all about bringing a little "ohm" into your life. In many ways, yoga is the perfect brain health exercise. As a physical activity, yoga supports your more vigorous aerobic workouts by building strength and stamina (not to dismiss the fact that yoga itself can be aerobic, depending on your practice). In addition, yoga helps build sustained focus, which we all need to learn and remember on a daily basis. Finally, yoga is a terrific resource for maintaining emotional balance, and can be used to reduce stress, anxiety and depressed mood, all of which may lower our everyday memory performance.

So try taking a 5 minute yoga break today. Kripalu, a center for yoga in Massachusetts, offers a series of such breaks you can download to your computer or other media player (www.kripalu.org). If you have time and are feeling even more ambitious, try an online yoga class from Yoga Today (www.yogatoday.com) or another online source. Consider looking for yoga classes in your area and making yoga part of your path to better brain health.

NOTES FOR DAY 15

DAY 15

Get Some Phone Game

How often during the day do you have 5 minutes when you are waiting with nothing to do? Stuck in traffic, waiting in a doctor's office, on hold for a conference call? Those breaks are the perfect time for a little brain game. Where might you find those games? On your phone, of course!

Games that we play on our phones or other mobile devices meet all my criteria for getting in a bit of brain skills training. Usually games we have to play against the clock, mobile based games get us to focus, think fast and think flexibly. Research has shown that by exercising these skills, which often can be challenged as we age, we can improve our performance in these areas.

So what are you waiting for? Pick up that phone and get some game! Don't have a game on your phone (or have no clue if you do or not?)? Most mobile service providers have games you can download to your phone for a minimal charge. Visit your provider's website for more information. Or if you are still clueless -- borrow a teenager!

NOTES FOR DAY 16

DAY 16

Learn the Symptoms of a Stroke

Today's tip teaches us about a serious threat to our brain's well-being – Stroke. Stroke is the leading cause of adult disability and third leading cause of death in the U.S.

Recently there have been tremendous advances in our ability to both prevent and treat for stroke. But you have to *know what to look for and be ready to act quickly*. I find that few folks really know the signs of a stroke - so let's learn them! This simple 3-step test, developed by researchers, is highly effective in identifying a stroke. If you suspect a stroke, try the following three things - if any of them are fail any of them, get to the ER as quickly as possible for an evaluation:

1. **Smile.** Ask the person to smile. Look for asymmetry (unevenness) in their facial expression (For example, if one corner of their mouth droops).

2. **Raise Both Arms.** Ask the person to raise both arms. Look for asymmetry in the height they can raise them.

3. **Repeat a Simple Sentence.** Ask the person to repeat a simple sentence, such as "No ifs, ands, or buts." Check for slurring or other disruption of speech.

Want to know more? Visit the National Stroke Association's website at www.stroke.org.

NOTES FOR DAY 17

DAY 17

Doodle!

Do you doodle? Many of us (including Bill Gates, former President Clinton and others) do. But did you realize that doodling might be good for your brain health?

Recent research suggests that doodling may help us attend, maintain focus, and remember more effectively. A study published in *Applied Cognitive Psychology* found that subjects assigned a doodling task not only did better when quizzed on what they were monitoring in a phone call, but also did 29% better than their non-doodling counterparts on a surprise memory test.

Why would something that improves attention matter to our memory? Attention is critical to acquisition, which is the first step of learning. Usually when we think we have forgotten something such as a name, in truth we simply weren't paying attention when we first learned it. As I often joke to my audiences, this is a "getting" not a "forgetting" problem. An activity like doodling, which improves attention, makes it more likely that you will acquire things that you want to recall.

So go ahead and doodle -- no need to feel guilty about it! If anyone asks, just tell them your doodle is helping your noodle (sorry, I just couldn't help it).

NOTES FOR DAY 18

DAY 18

Get Verbal

Today's tip gives you a chance to expand your mind by expanding your vocabulary.

Research has demonstrated that intellectual activities may reduce our risk for serious memory impairment. For example, one study at the Rush University Medical Center in Illinois found that folks who reported participating regularly in such activities had an associated reduced risk for memory impairment of approximately 26%. While no one knows why intellectual engagement seems to have protective benefits for the brain, one prevailing theory suggests that such activities give us "cognitive reserve" which provides a cushion so that symptoms of memory impairment will be delayed.

What better way to get your mind engaged than by expanding your vocabulary? Building your word skills can really make you think and is a great prep for word games, writing, and other intellectual challenges. Besides, this is a tip that is fast, free, and fun.

There are some great online resources for getting more out of your vocabulary. Try www.freerice.com (and donate rice to the World Hunger Program at the same time) or sign up on one of several sites to receive a "Word of the Day."

NOTES FOR DAY 19

DAY 19

Juggle!

Have you ever tried juggling? And not just your schedule? Today's tip is all about getting you and your brain back in the juggling game.

Why does juggling make our list? Complex motor integration activities such as juggling have been shown to increase brain volume and improve everyday memory performance. Researchers in Germany found that juggling increased volume in their subjects' brain white matter. Another group, looking at the impact of computer based dance games on everyday intellectual performance, found that folks with the smoothest moves scored higher on tests of verbal memory. Such activities boost brain health by getting us to move and forcing us to focus and think about what we are doing. and – best of all! – they rate very high on the "fun" factor.

Chances are you may have tried juggling at one time in your life, only to give it up as too difficult. Today is your chance to give juggling another shot. Start with one or two balls or scarves (scarves may be a bit easier at first) then slowly work your way up to three. Want more direction? You can easily find instructional help on the internet.

NOTES FOR DAY 20

DAY 20

Hug Five People

Here's a tip that will move your mind and your heart. Today's brain booster asks you to give 5 people a hug.

Why is today's tip about getting more huggable? Studies have shown that folks who are more socially engaged have an associated reduced risk for memory impairment. In one recent study, researchers at the Harvard School of Public Health found that participants who reported lower levels of social interaction were significantly more likely to show memory problems after 6 years than their more social peers. Maintaining our emotional ties can also reduce our risk for emotional distress, depression and stress, all of which have been linked to an increase in daily memory problems and dementia risk.

So go out there and get your hugs going. Hopefully this one won't prove too hard for you to do! Just keep in mind that those hugs aren't only good for your soul, they're good for your brain.

Happy hugs!

NOTES FOR DAY 21

DAY 21

Do a Sentence Scramble

Verbal word games can be addictive. Many of us love these puzzles, and they are without doubt the most popular kind of game among my clients.

How are word games good for our brains? Such activities keep us intellectually engaged by getting us to "stretch" our thinking. Unlike timed activities, which offer us a different kind of challenge, word games (and puzzles, board games and the like) grab our attention, get us to make new connections, and give us the chance to think outside of our mind's box.

Here's a word game you may not have played before -- Sentence Scramble. It's a quick, fun word game that does all of the above and gives your creativity a boost as well. How do you play Sentence Scramble? First, take a newspaper, magazine or book and turn to a random page. Next, select a paragraph (any one will do) and go through it. Take every fifth word from that paragraph and write it down, until you have a list of 8-10 words. Now you are ready to play! Take that list of word and make up a sentence, using only those words -- the quirkier and sillier your sentence, the better.

NOTES FOR DAY 22

DAY 22

Wear Your Watch Upside Down

Today's tip will make time fly. Give your brain a little stretch each time you check your watch by wearing your watch upside down. This subtle change won't take much effort to do, but will force your brain to think out of its comfort zone in making sense of time gone a bit topsy-turvy. These kinds of "neurobic" activities (a phrase coined by Dr. Lawrence Katz) may seem fun and simple, yet are a terrific way to challenge our brain's flexibility and routine.

Like this exercise? Keep it going all week!

Have a good time!

NOTES FOR DAY 23

DAY 23

Meditate for 5 Minutes

Today's tip focuses on the "soul" side of brain health. You may not think of meditation as "brain healthy" but it may be one of the best things you can do for your brain.

A simple way to think about meditation is the practice of being still within one's self. Meditation offers many benefits to brain health. Meditation is a perfect way to build attention, as it trains us to hold focus. It can also help us more effectively manage pain, stress, and emotional distress, all of which can detract from daily memory performance. Finally, there is emerging interest in the physiological benefits of meditation, with some studies suggesting that meditation may offer a way to target different centers of the brain to maintain function.

To get started, set aside 5 minutes to sit in a quiet spot in your house, at a time when you will not be interrupted. Get comfortably seated (on the floor or on a chair). Now, just be there, in that moment, observing your breath. As thoughts come to your mind (as they will), notice them and then just let them go. If you need help passing by those thoughts, here are two methods I have found helpful. First, just comment to yourself "everything passes" and then let the thought go. Or try my yoga teacher's approach -- as the thoughts come, think to yourself "blah, blah, blah" (which is really the "noise" those thoughts "make" after all) and let them go.

NOTES FOR DAY 24

DAY 24

Write a Haiku

What better way to begin your day than with a mind stretching exercise certain to be poetry to your ears? Writing Haiku is a wonderful way to get out of your "boxed in" brain and challenge yourself to think differently and creatively.

Haiku is an ancient Japanese form of verse, dating back centuries in its origin. Haiku is known for its simple form, which requires a pattern of 5 syllables, 7 syllables and 5 syllables. Classical haiku also makes use of images that are seasonal and sensory in nature.

While I am by no means a Haiku expert, here's my try at today's tip to get you going --

> She sat at her desk
> The snow glistened in the sun
> The tree shivered cold.

For more about the art of Haiku, take a look online at one of the many instructional sites.

Happy Haiku!

NOTES FOR DAY 25

DAY 25

Do Something Kind

Today's tip has you help others and at the same time help yourself (or your brain). Studies have shown that folks who volunteer have the added benefit of better overall health. In one study from the Johns Hopkins University Medical Center, older adults who served as volunteer reading tutors at a local elementary school improved on measures of cognitive well-being as well. In addition to giving us an opportunity to "do good," volunteering our time gives us the chance to stay intellectually and socially engaged, which have both been associated with reducing our risk for memory impairment.

Take a little time today to do something kind. Shovel your neighbor's walk (great physical exercise as well), pay an extra compliment to your teen, talk to someone who looks a bit lonely. Not only is it good for your brain, it's good for you.

NOTES FOR DAY 26

DAY 26

Reconnect with a Long-Lost Friend

All of us have friends from the past with whom we have lost touch over the years. Today's tip offers you the chance to reconnect with one of those long lost buddies.

Why rekindle that friendship? Research has shown that higher levels of social engagement are associated with reduced risk for memory loss. Also, being with others gives us a great "skills" workout, as you really can't be social without staying focused, thinking fast and keeping your mind nimble. Staying social also exposes us to different experiences or ways of thinking, which is great for our intellectual engagement. Finally, our brain benefits from the "intangible" side of staying social, by lowering our risk for emotional distress.

In our busy day-to-day lives, it is altogether too easy to lose track of friends whose company we really enjoy. So spend some time today finding that long lost pal. Use the internet (Facebook and Google are great tools for this), dig out an old phone book or alumni directory. Call or write, reconnect, and make a plan to stay in touch.

NOTES FOR DAY 27

DAY 27

Play Solitaire

Today's tip is to play solitaire. There are many forms of this card game, several of which you may remember from childhood. Why play solitaire? Card games like solitaire give us an easy and familiar way to "challenge" our brain just a bit each day. As we've seen, staying intellectually engaged in this way may give our brains some added protection against memory loss. In addition, games like solitaire can be relaxing and ease emotional distress.

So spend a few minutes today digging out that deck of cards and playing a few rounds of your favorite Solitaire game. You can even play versions of the game, such as Free Cell, online. Need a refresher course on the game? Just look for directions for various Solitaire games online to get started. A little Solitaire can be a great way to pass the time and give our brains a little boost.

NOTES FOR DAY 28

DAY 28

Spend 10 Minutes Organizing Your Desk

Today's tip will help clear some clutter from your life. Folks who are organized remember better. Why? They have mastered one of the best memory secrets - memory tools.

Organizational strategies are the best way we can remind ourselves of things we have to do or places we have to be. Think of organizational strategies as essential ingredients of your memory improvement program.

To get started, spend 10 minutes today organizing your desk. Get rid of what is non-essential. File away what you can. Look over how your desk is organized and consider whether it works for you. Can you think of a better way to put it all together? Just think how great it will be to come back tomorrow to your newly organized workspace.

For more on why organizational strategies are critical to a good memory, take a look at my book **Total Memory Workout: 8 Easy Steps for Maximum Memory Fitness** for organizational tools guaranteed to boost your brain power.

NOTES FOR DAY 29

DAY 29

Parlez vous Francais?

Today's tip asks you to listen to the world a bit differently. Give your brain a stretch today by tuning in to a foreign radio station. Listening to another language -- and trying to understand it -- is another slightly out of the ordinary and terrific way we can challenge our minds to stay intellectually active.

You can easily find foreign radio stations in your area by exploring around the dial. Or tune in to ones online. Try a station that airs in a language you studied in high school, or one that you've always wanted to learn. Who knows, today's tip may even inspire you to finally sign up for that language course you've always wanted to take, making today's "brain stretch" even more long lasting.

A bientot!

NOTES FOR DAY 30

| |
| |
| |
| |
| |
| |
| |
| |
| |
| |
| |
| |
| |
| |
| |
| |
| |
| |
| |

DAY 30

List 10 Ways Your Brain is Great

Today is the final day of our *30 Days to Better Brain Health* Plan. As a way of wrapping up the terrific work you've done to boost your memory and build better brain power, take a few minutes and list 10 ways in which your brain is totally awesome.

Why take the time to reflect on our brain's strengths? I find that as we grow older and worry about memory loss, we tend to lose sight of all the really amazing things our brains do on a daily basis. Our brains are responsible for everything from keeping us awake (and getting us to sleep) to maintaining our senses, helping us speak, letting us love, and giving us pleasure in the experience of new things, each and every day. So its important to take the time and think about what our brains do well, for a change -- and I bet that you will quickly complete that list of 10 items.

I hope that you've enjoyed the 30 Days to Better Brain Health program and learning how to boost your brain power!

Here's to many happy memories!

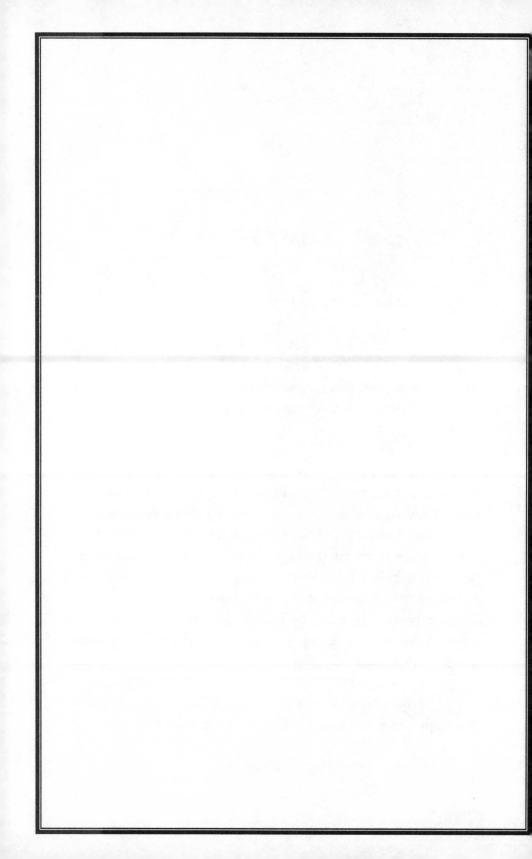

For more information about the Total Brain Health® program and Dr. Green, please visit:

www.totalbrainhealth.com

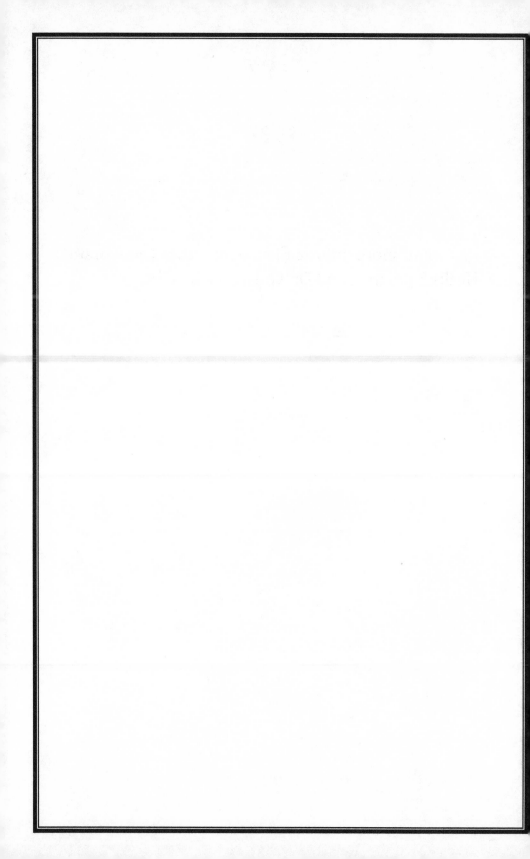

CPSIA information can be obtained
at www.ICGtesting.com
Printed in the USA
BVHW032341231019
561881BV00002B/252/P